Refugees' healthcare services through comprehensive Primary Health Care

A "Refugee Friendly Clinic"

An initiative of the Department of Family Medicine and Primary HealthCare

Ghent University- Belgium

Dr. Ahmad Khalid Zurmati, MD - 2017

The backbone point was how barriers should be managed and how we could be able to solve the problems and find solutions to the problems; it was nothing except the best leadership, good communication and evidence based healthcare services and we named it "Barriers Breakers".

Contains

1. Acknowledgment

I would like to express my deepest appreciation to all those who provided me such opportunity to work for this project. A special gratitude I give to Prof. Dr. Jan De Maeseneer MD-PhD whose contribution in stimulating idea and his encouragement, helped me to write this technical report.

Furthermore I would like to acknowledge with much appreciation the crucial role of the staff in Project Ponton who gave me praise to finish this technical report. My special thanks goes to Dr. Peter Decat, MD-PhD who invested his full effort to guide the Ponton team in a daily base toward achieving the goal. Last but not least many thanks goes to our dedicated nurse, Ms. Klaartje Dossche, who provided me administrative support.

Dr. Zurmati A K, MD

Ghent, March 2017

2. Abbreviations

CLB	Students Guidance Centre (Centra voor Leerlingenbegeleiding)
CPHC	Comprehensive Primary HealthCare
GP	General Practitioner
ICPC	International Classification of Primary Care
ICD	International Classification of Diseases
FEDASIL	Federal Agency for Reception of Asylum Seekers/ Belgium
FGM	Female Genital Mutilation
LGBT	An initialism that stands for lesbian, gay, bisexual, and transgender
PC	Primary Care
PHC	Primary Health Care
PTSD	Post Traumatic Stress Disorder
TB	Tuberculosis
UNHCR	United Nations High Commissioner for Refugees, also known as the UN Refugee Agency
WHO	World Health Organisation

3. Preface

By: Prof. Dr. Jan De Maeseneer, MD-PhD

This report by Dr. Ahmed Khalid Zurmati, a Medical Doctor and refugee from Afghanistan, represents a seminal paper on refugees and health.

The report starts from the organization of comprehensive health care with family physicians/general practitioners, nurses, psychologists, social workers,... in the clinic on the "Ponton – RENO", and widens the scope to the socio-political, ethical and cultural context of health care for refugees. The merits of an interprofessional approach in these circumstances are clearly illustrated, especially when it comes to deal with mental health and severe conditions like PTSD (Post-Traumatic Stress Disorder).

But this document is more than just a report. It reflects the power of solidarity that originates from an open mind, that does not want to build walls, but that builds bridges. Bridges from the PONTON to the quay and from there to the community. Schools, local citizens, socio-cultural organizations, volunteers, city agencies, civil society organizations, private not-for-profit agencies and private companies, all work together to create a warm, human context. This energetic warmth may inspire us all, so that we do not forget that solidarity creates hope for a better life and a better future, especially for those most in need, for those who have to leave their country because of violence and war.

Thanks to all who made this unique experience on the "Ponton – RENO" and in the city of Ghent possible and especially to the team that worked on the Ponton. Thanks to the city of Ghent that demonstrated that there is an alternative and the name of that alternative is "solidarity".

Thanks to Dr. Khalid Zurmati to create for us through this report, the opportunity to become part of this unique human experience.

Prof. Jan De Maeseneer, MD, PhD, (Hon) FRCGP.
Head Department of Family Medicine and Primary Health Care.
Ghent University.

3.1 Preface

By: Prof. Dr. Ignaas Devisch, PhD

We are proud to present you the final report of the Refugees' healthcare services based on an initiative from our Department of Family Medicine and Primary HealthCare at Ghent University. The initiative known in layman's term as 'the Ponton' was created to cope with the health needs and challenges of newcomers and asylum seekers in Belgium.

The Ponton took care with emergencies, gave first aid based on best evidence and coordinated consultation with appropriate referral and transportation to the second or tertiary healthcare services. Next to that, the vocational training offered to GP's at Belgian universities, enabled them to provide a higher level of comprehensive and continuous health care in a special family practice setting of the Ponton. Only last year, the GP's were able to held more than two thousand consultation in a residential place of 250 diverse inhabitants.

This report presents an overview of past activities and results. We were able to help people in difficult circumstances and a context of fragility and uncertainty. Taking care of people is the most basic attitude one may expect from medicine. But taking care of people in difficult circumstances includes more than doing your job. It asks for engagement and ethical commitment. Hopefully, our primary care has supported the asylum seekers in their process integration and feeling welcome in our society.

Dr. A. Khalid Zurmati has done an excellent job and I thank him for writing this very readable report and his engagement.

Prof. Dr. Ignaas Devisch, PhD
Department of Family Medicine and Primary HealthCare
Ethics and Philosophy of Medicine

4. Summary

Purpose – This report presents an overview of the past activities and main results of the "Project Ponton" which was aimed to cope with the health needs of asylum seekers[6] in the city of Ghent in Belgium. The main objectives were to take care of their health as a basic of their human rights through comprehensive healthcare delivery.

Design – This technical paper prepared based on reporting on inputs, outputs, outcome and the process itself.

Findings – Professionalism and commitment, respect and admire psycho-socio-cultural aspects of individuals, and an active multi-sectoral collaboration were the key factors for project success.

Implementing the real Comprehensive Primary Healthcare (CPHC) model in a temporary asylum seekers center isn't an easy job. Consequently by building a consortium alike "Ponton consortium" which was comprised of the majority required stakeholders of a CPHC, we were able to play as a CPHC in real in an inappropriate infrastructure. the multidisciplinary team of family doctors, nurses, physiotherapists and psychologists were recruited among local care providers, acquainted with the local health care system and committed to deliver the best possible care to those people in need. This local embedment greatly facilitated collaboration with and referral to local health care organizations. Moreover the team could – for more refugee-specific problems - rely on the help of an Afghan physician with refugee background who gave support especially in handling psychosocial issues and mental health problems. The added value of his engagement in the team surpassed largely the purely language-related issues as his lived experience also contributed to an improved cultural sensitive interaction between health care providers and residents.

The role of the nurses was of crucial importance. They were the first point of contact. They evaluated the demand, gave advise, started a treatment, referred to the GP and provided follow up care. Due to their professionalism, commitment and personal approach they gained trust and respect from the residents which contributed largely to the successful health outcomes.

In the many critical and delicate cases there was close interdisciplinary consultation which resulted in a consented and polyvalent approach of complex problems. The nurses often acted as intermediaries between the parties.

Lastly, the engagement of local organizations (infant care, centers for pupils' counseling, social welfare, buddy project, psychiatric crisis team, homecare etc.) was a tremendous advantage and contributed to long term solutions for complex cases.

The Ponton experience bears witness that local family doctors are very well positioned to coordinate the care for refugees and asylum-seekers. The perspective of family medicine is indispensable for adjusting health care systems to respond to the changed health needs concurring with the current migration crisis.

Report limitations – Due to unavailability of Pricare Data for the time being we couldn't able to do in deep epidemiological data analysis. By obtaining of Pricare data in the near by future, we will conduct series of epidemiological studies to explore more possibilities.

Practical implications – Report realized that to shape a "Refugee Friendly Clinic", we need equity in healthcare delivery through presenting the best policies along with enhancing transcultural skills of professionals or recruiting professionals from a Refugee background.

Social implications – A predictable social impact of the similar projects will be fastening newcomers integration process by responding to their psychosocial needs.

Value – This technical paper presents that to protect human rights of newcomers there are commitment of health professionals which can be endorsed by commitment of politicians.

Keywords: Ponton, Refugee, Human Rights, Newcomers, Pricare, Primary care, Integration, Equity, Health.

Type: Technical Paper/Report

5. Pre Ponton

15 February 2016

Far away from politics yet not far from ignorance of three words: immigrants, shelter and health services were the main disquiets of professionals who devoted in the process of responding to the Hippocrates's oat. After several meetings with stakeholders, finally I, Prof. Dr. Jan De Maeseneer and two lady doctors got the chance to visit the Ponton[c] for the first time. We had an appointment with director of the Ponton' in the Regakaai of Ghent city at 1:00 PM sharp, but due to unavailability of exact GPS address, we reached there at 1:15 PM, anyway a sunny day accompanying a world known dedicated Professor, which is "Primary Healthcare", is in his heart and spirit, was a privilege . On the other hand, visiting "Ponton" after mass media's controversy was another excitement and heart beating feeling along with an unknown anxiety. Finally we reached there and I saw a different picture which was totally opposite to the media's controversy. I along with my family do have a five months living experience in an asylum center here in Belgium, I couldn't compare both centers from quality point of view thus "Ponton" was built as a very sophisticated residential place for about 300 prisoners along with all basic facilities in which now it has been transformed to a new residential place alike river touched hotel closed to a big city.

We are a dedicated team of health and medical professionals, affiliated with the Ghent University along with collaboration of community and volunteers. We have developed a clinic plan in a unique place of Ghent to serve newly arriving Asylum seekers[6] in the city of Ghent. We are a divers team of physicians and health care professionals with expertise in refugee care who can communicate and offer initial assessment and medical services in different and divers languages and cultures.

Taken all above into account, we had more concerns about the administration and logistic part of Ponton[c] because it's the first time ever in history of Ghent that a commercial security company is managing a unique humanitarian project and get an outsourced not for profit project.

Preparedness means investment; Project Ponton[c] was not just a unique project to show our solidarity to the newcomers; but it became a fantastic lesson learned about the current situation of refugees in Belgium!6. Project Brief Report

After the recent storm of newcomers in Europe, an enormous advocacy of individuals and academics made a decision that Municipality of Ghent in Belgium may take and lodge a group of newcomers, and GPs[a] have to register clinical data of Asylum seekers[6] in PriCare software and could provide health care delivery inside the center on a daily base. Department of Family Medicine and Primary HealthCare of Ghent Universit[4] decided to start a pilot project in a new Asylum seekers[6] center through a consortium cooperation named "Ponton-Reno[20]. Avoiding discrimination on the grounds of providing equitable healthcare for all, patient's privacy and keeping their medical record safely, were the main objectives of this intervention. Based on the current Belgian laws, individual's immigration status does not affect their eligibility for free primary care and emergency healthcare services.

The way training provided to the GPs[a] here in Belgian universities, enabled GPs[a] to provide a high level of comprehensive and continuous health care in a special family practice setting of Pontonc[c].

Dealing with emergencies, giving proper first aid based on best evidence, coordinating consultation with appropriate referral and transportation to the second or tertiary healthcare services, were GPs[a] and other health and medical staff endeavor have contributed to a quality way of practice. During past one year, GPs[a] in Ponton[c] were able to held more than two thousand consultation in a residential place of 250 diverse inhabitants.

Effective management of common diseases in the Ponton[c] by family physicians and nurses either presenting with common or wide range of common/ unusual symptoms was a tremendous experience. The team was able to take more than two hundred histories and general checkups along with doing laboratory examinations of common and sexual transmitted diseases to all inhabitants. Acknowledging the importance of comprehensive care with continuity, using a holistic approach was another focus of Ponton's comprehensive family medicine healthcare delivery.

Effective communication with Asylum seekers[6], their families, colleagues and other health care worker, and community; by recruiting multilingual professional staff as well as staff by refugee background brought to the project a lot of assets, especially in psychosocial issues and when treating mental health problems. By applying knowledge of behavioral and social sciences in the patient management plan, respecting the autonomy, dignity and rights of the patient/ family; the Project Ponton[c] discovered more soft and sound tools of patient-doctor relation, which are all based on respecting divers culture believes and control of diversity. Promoting health, organizing preventive care measures and supporting the national health programs; were defined as GPs[a] and nurses' preventive responsibilities which they were able to make and provide different brochures in different languages for prevention of Bed Buds, Scabies, Sexual transmitted diseases, etc.

Practicing cost-effective management with knowledge of health economics and following the FEDASIL[15] guideline was essential for practice in Project Ponton[c]. Above mentioned practice was tearful sometimes, because of uncertainty or denying of treatment of some cases through FEDASIL[15].

Run-through managerial skills including medical record keeping, auditing, coordination within the health service system and recognizing the importance of quality assurance; through keeping of hard and soft copies specially by introducing PriCare software in an Asylum seekers' center in Belgium contributed to a remarkable outcome and easy data collection instrument. By critical appraisal of medical information on refugee's health. GPs[a] in Ponton[c], managed more evidenced based medicine.

In conclusion last but not least all family physicians and other team members were committed to the Self-directed lifelong learning and continuous professional development to prepare more for influential humanitarian assistance. The core issue of medical ethics and law with ability to handle medico-legal issues and maintain professional ethical standards, were of ground rules for family medicine practice in the Ponton[c].

All above process brought a fine, easy and ethical accepted line of a comprehensive primary health care delivery manner to a needy community of Asylum seekers which is in turn may encourage a soft, healthy and short time period of integration process of newcomers in the society.

The Ponton team tried to think about different research methods to undertake needs-based research on refugees health. By extracting anonymous PriCare software data, they assumed a serial of related issues studies needed, they planned to do research on Refugees Health.

....

a-General practitioners , b- Federal Agency for the Reception od Asylum seekers, c- Name of Asylum Seekers Center in Ghent

7. Background

War and climate change is widely projected to cause substantial increases in the scale of human population movement in coming decades. Forecasts predict that by around midcentury tens of millions to 250 million people in response to the effects of war and climate change vary from (Boano et al. 2008, Brown 2007, UNHCR 2009). In 2015 over one million people arrived in Europe (by sea), mostly originating from Syria, Afghanistan, Iraq and African countries. The estimate by Myers in 2002 that climate change[2]will cause up to an additional 200 million environmental refugees by 2050 is now widely accepted. Many of those who reached Europe across the sea or via other itineraries, continue to face threats to their health and security. While some of them suffer from chronic medical conditions that stay un-attended, others are pregnant without access to prenatal care. Many of the refugees and Asylum seekers[6] are children, some with respiratory infections, others suffer from mental trauma related to the conflict and prosecution they are fleeing from. The fear of repatriation or detention and bureaucratic hurdles makes them potentially doubt about seeking healthcare.

Refugees and Asylum seekers, who have access to some kind of healthcare in Europe are also suffering from several challenges. Whilst some of these challenges are not related to their medical conditions, such as language barriers and cultural differences, others are medical or public health related issues. By 2050 Germany, France and United Kingdom will have approximately 80 million people as a consequence of immigration. Immigration is not easy to forecast. In past three years 2015-2017, Germany hosted about one million immigrants mostly from war turned countries: Syria, Afghanistan and Iraq plus a silent wave of immigrants from Africa.

8. Refugees and the Belgian healthcare system

In Belgium, the registered Asylum seekers[6] and refugees are entitled to Belgian healthcare. We explain how to have access to the healthcare services in Belgium when somebody has Asylum seeker or a refugee status.

Based on international humanitarian and UN's agreed laws and regulations, in Belgium registered Asylum seekers[6] will enjoy access to health care services; these services are paid by FEDASI[15] and will not cover all care services, the limitation of payable healthcare services to Asylum seekers[6] are controlled by the PHC (Primary Health Care) system based on FEDASIL's guideline.

In case of illness, Asylum seekers[6] will be entitled to see a Family Physician (Huisarts).

In emergency cases Asylum seekers[6] will be introduced by Asylum seekers[6] centers authorities to a hospital for care and FEDASIL[15] will reimburse the care cost to the hospital, health facility or individual providers.

In Belgium priority conditions to address in the Asylum centers are as following:

- General checkup and medical history taking

- Common Mental Health Disorders (including PTSD and depression)

- Vaccination for Preventable Diseases

- Skin conditions (including Scabies and Cellulitis)

- Tuberculosis

- Sexual and Physical Violence

- Referral to specialized care (mostly in emergency cases)

Recognized refugees who are living and working in Belgium are covered by the Belgian healthcare system. The Belgian healthcare system is one of the best in Europe but you have to have access to social security benefits to use it.

Belgian health insurance

The Belgian healthcare system is divided into public and private sectors, with fees payable in both, funded by a combination of social security contributions and tax money. With mandatory health insurance, patients are free to choose their own medical professionals and places of treatment. Patients generally pay costs upfront and are reimbursed a proportion of the charges for medical and dental fees, hospital care and treatment, maternity costs and drug prescriptions through their health insurance fund (mutualiteit / ziekenfonds)[1]. Some alternative treatments are also reimbursable (through the complementary health care insurance) if they are carried out by a qualified physician. Many people top up their cover with private insurance to get a full refund of (almost) all medical costs.

Doctors work in public and/or private settings. Dentists are almost all private. Hospitals and clinics are private and usually managed by universities, religious organizations, or social entrepreneurs.
Healthcare providers for Asylum seekers6 and refugees mostly follow the FEDASIL's guideline for the medical services[6.]

9. Ponton's medical team

The medical team of Ponton[c] as part of consortium for refugees care systematically pursued the ethical values and provided quality services to meet their mission to protect, promote, and improve the health of all Asylum seekers[6] and refugees in Ponton[c] through comprehensive primary healthcare by means of equitable access to care, community participation, devotion to social determinants of health, intersectoral cooperation and health advocacy.

9.1Objectives

The team was there to meet the following objectives:

- To identify health problems of newcomers in Ponton[c]

- To identify factors that affects health in Ponton[c]

- Act as a stimulus for making positive health changes in Ponton[c]

- To act as a stimulus for inter-sectoral and community action

- To identify new needs and indicators for refugees' health

- To inform the public, politicians, professionals and policy makers about matters that affect the health of refugees in an easily understandable way.

The main purpose of Ponton's health report is to stimulate action to improve refugees health by:

- Providing accurate, unbiased and independent information about the refugees' health

- Providing accurate, unbiased and independent information about the determinants of health in the Ponton[c] as an example.

- Inspiring all relevant groups to take action to improve health of refugees in asylum centers.

- Conducting related researches based on acceptable ethical issues

10. Outlines

This final report is a glimpse report of the Project Ponton[c] through comprehensive Primary Healthcare services have been prepared using the anonymous daily records, FEDASIL[15] guideline, official e-mail correspondences between Prof. Dr. Jan De Maeseneer, Dr. A. Khalid Zurmati, Dr. Peter Decat, and other medical team members. We also went through official domestic and international agreements toward refugees' health, all above will cover the following:

1. Inputs, processes, outputs and outcomes of the project (e.g. what was achieved and how and by who).

2. The stakeholder (consortium) involved and the nature and the impact of partnering activities (especially in relation of ongoing efforts/impacts).

3. Enablers and barriers to the work/implementation of the project and how barriers were managed.

4. Provision of hard or electronic copies of any relevant documentation produced (e.g. medical record).

5. Statement around whether proposed projects effectively/efficiently achieved the anticipated outputs and outcomes.

6. Advice on sustainability especially in relation to the following types of issues:

- Organizations Infrastructure (fit with goals and cultures)

- Staff (Training and involvement, Attitudes ,Senior leaders, Clinical leaders)

- Process (Monitoring progress , Adaptability , Credibility of evidence, Benefits beyond helping patients).

10.1. Input:

Fortunately we had many promising and dedicating resources that contributed in our unique ever project for Refugees' healthcare services, such as following :

10.1.1 Funding:

The core budget that was provided by FEDASIL[15], besides other health governmental health organizations brought additional resources in a very sophisticated manner. Our volunteer's, contribution especially as buddies for psychosocial wellbeing is an unforgettable community contribution. We will never forget community's gift in kind which was put a fine impression on refugees minds.

10.1.2. Staff:

Mostly the Ponton[c] was staffed by G4S a private company as FEDASIL[15] contractor; in particular Ponton[c] clinic had one and half nursing staff hired by G4S, and four Family physicians, four psychologists coordinated through Ghent University. Out of the day hours on call doctors from Community Health Centers were onother asset which is more cost effective than ambulance service.

10.1.3. Time:

Time input for clinic was 38 hours per week as regular hours, but 24 hours for emergency through governmental healthcare services.

Availability of at least one medical staff during the official day hours was an obligation.

Four regular days of consultation per week through family physicians and availability of a dedicated multilingual physician as on call physician(24/7) was an asset for the Clinic.

10.1.4. Equipment:
The clinic was located in the ground floor just in the right side of Ponton[c] entrance, a waiting room, two consultation rooms and a procedure and pharmacy room.

The equipments were basic including two examination beds, all necessary examination tools, an emergency drug shelf, two PCs along with installed Pricare software and internet connection, communication tools e.g. two sets of digital telephones and walky-talkies.

10.1.5. Contribution of other organizations in kind or volunteer:
Many volunteer organizations were around and offered their skills and contribution , especially Kind&Gezin(Child and family), school health services (CLB), NGOs for psychosocial wellbeing of newcomers.

10.2. Output:
The Medical team members were able to provide services as follows:

Regular check-up and intake, medical examination, diagnosis and treatment, epidemiological monitoring, monthly statistical report, developing of health promotion measures and tools, study designs, Pricare coding (using ICPC-2-classification), writing articles , participation in the education of medical students, developing of standards and guidelines in different languages.

Starting from the quote "Evidence based healthcare is a must", Project Ponton[c] indicators were dealing with the following:

— Total number of consultations handled

— Total number of referrals to secondary level healthcare services

— Total number of vaccines administrated

— Total number of the psychological consultations with patients performed

- Total number children were seen through the Child &Family agency

- Total number of school children seen by CLB (for primary and secondary school children)

- Total number of medical emergency cases

- Total number of patients were referred to physiotherapy

- Total number of pregnant women were cared

- Total number of LGBT were cared

- Total number of FGM were cared

- Health promotion leaflets in different languages were prepared and distributed.

- Research opportunities were made.

Table 1: Global figures of the care provided at the Ponton:

Total inhabitants	Average number of		Total consultations
	Patients week	consultation per	mostly registered & coded in Pricare
250	40		2080

Above table shows an average number of consultations/visits with a physician per person per year in Ponton[c] which was 8.32 visits per person with a family physician.

The average number of consultations with a physician per person per year includes consultations at the physician's office, in the patient's home, or in out-patient departments in hospitals or ambulatory health care centers. It excludes consultations/visits during a treatment in a hospital or similar institution as part of in-patient or day care patient care.

Among the EU Member States there is a wide range in the distribution of the number of consultations to physicians. In Cyprus and Sweden the annual average was less than 3.0 consultations per inhabitant per year, with this average ranging between 4.1 and 8.7 consultations in most other Member States. Although Germany, the Czech Republic, Slovakia and Hungary were above this range.

Between 2009 and 2014, the average number of consultations increased in seven of the 19 EU Member States for which data are available (see Figure 1 for data availability)[7]

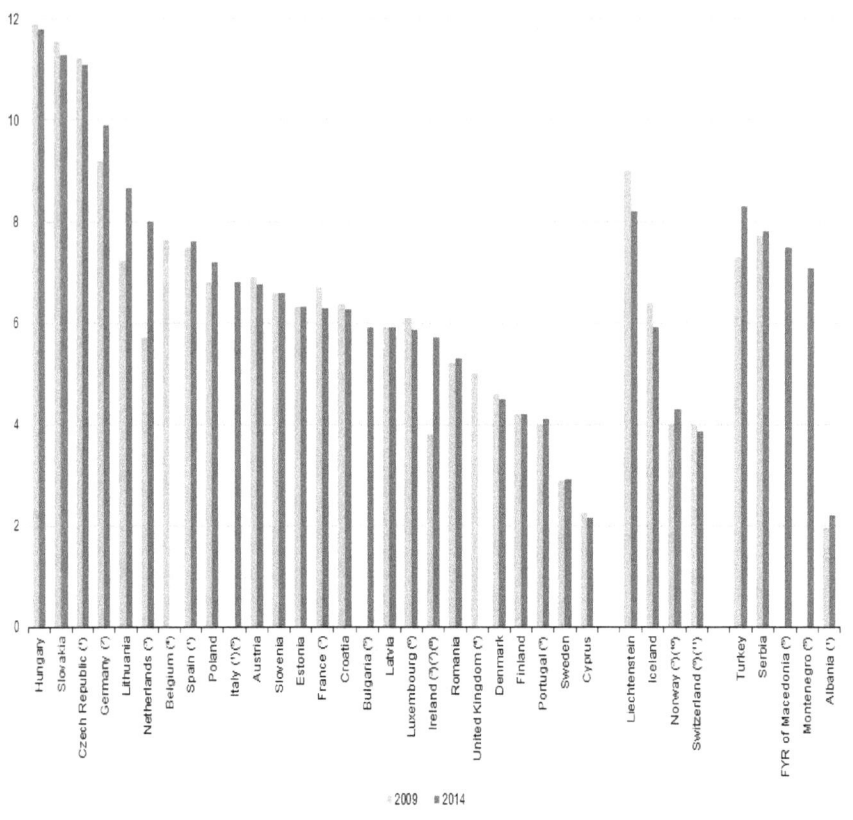

Note: Greece and Malta: not available.
(¹) 2013 instead of 2014.
(²) Definition differs.
(³) Break in series.
(⁴) 2014: not available.
(⁵) 2009: not available.
(⁶) 2014: estimate.
(⁷) 2010 instead of 2009.
(⁸) 2015 instead of 2014.
(⁹) 2012 instead of 2014.
(¹⁰) 2009: estimate.
(¹¹) 2007 instead of 2009.

Fig 1: Average number of consultations per inhabitant per year, according to country comparison 2009-2014

The refferals in Ponton to specialty care were limited , in accordance with the FEDASIL[15] guideline. The total number of referals except emergency cases were 104 which was 5% of all consultations per year.

Table 2: Immunity, status of inhabitants for selected infectious disease:

Positive Anti-HAV	Positive HBs Ag	Positive Anti-HCV	Positive Anti- HIV	Positive T. Pallidum
93.54%	12.9%	6.45%	6.45%	6.45%

TB and Malaria: Two TB cases were diagnosed and they were under close monitoring of TB institute, recently declared free of sickness.

Two Malaria cases were diagnosed and patients received Antimalarial treatment.

Vaccination

About 50% of inhabitant received their vaccination , mostly second round of their vaccinations after initial shot in Brussels on the time of their Asylum appeal.

Vaccines that were administrated to newcomers namely were as the following:

Polio, Measles, rubella, Pertussis, Diphtheria, Tetanus, Tuberculosis and Hepatitis B

Table 3: Chronic conditions

Chronic Diseases	Number of Pts under observation & treatment
Multimorbidity	8
Diabetes Mellitus	6
Heart disease	3
Hypertension	8

11. Outbreaks/ Interventions

During the one year time of the project, we were able to diagnose several Scabies cases and they were immediately treated. All diagnosed cases were imported cases from other residential places of Asylum seekers[6].

Two Malaria Vivax cases had been diagnosed and already received treatment. It was probably an imported case.

12. Psychosocial services

Asylum seekers[6] and refugees often present with complex needs as a result of post-traumatic experiences including following torture, rape, violent incidents, loss of family members, job, home, culture, lack of recognition in society. All have concerns about loved ones left back in homeland or missing. Once in the host country, Asylum seekers[6] and refugees often suffer from high levels of anxiety about the complex asylum process in the host country. They worry about accommodation, money, education, access to legal advice, detention, fear of deportation or destitution, homelessness and the most important issue of finding a reasonable job as per their smallest satisfaction.

Ponton[c] Psychosocial Service, coordinated by Prof. Ilse Derluyn (Ghent University) recognized that an individual asylum seeker's mental health is an important factor in their life. During one year the team was able to meet needy patients about 350 times by our dedicated four psychologists. beside our Psychosocial Service volunteers were also dedicated to provide GroupWise or individualized, person centered psychosocial support and services.

Psychosocial Service at Ponton[c] assisted the management team in supporting individual's needs of its residents during their short-term stay. Pontonc's Psychosocial Service assisted Asylum seekers[6] inside the campus as well as identifying, providing, or using outside resources to support their psychosocial needs, including those with post-traumatic stress disorder, anxiety, depression, addictions, and other mental health and individualized conditions.

The time limited therapeutic support (as per offered by our clinic and colleagues) in the form of early wellbeing assessments and work with individuals to address the psycho social needs of Asylum seekers[6] and refugees to reduce distress is an appreciable task.

13. Health promotion:

We were able to control the spreading of scabies through different audio-visual instruments and took preventive measures for the future diagnosis, treatment and prevention of scabies in the Reno- Ponton[c].

Developed and translated reading materials (English, Dari, Persian, Pashto):

Bedbugs, Scabies, Hepatitis B&C, Personal Hygiene. All were distributed among Asylum seekers6.

14. Training and participation in medical students education

- Many students in groups or individually participated in our routine activities.

- A group of guest students from Uzbekistan visited from Ponton's medical services.

- A number of educative articles about Hepatitis B, Vit.D deficiency among the newcomers and Refugees' health were written and will be published soon.

15. Community Outcomes

Community outcomes are the particular future or state of affairs valued by each community.

We tried to identify and define community outcomes, which was encouraged by Ghent Health Council directly and indirectly to inform central government and others about community needs,

A key concept in this process of understanding for the communities and setting goals for achieving community outcomes is 'well-being'. The way well-being is defined locally depends on factors such as personal values, cultures, social norms and world view, but it generally encompasses secure livelihood, health, safety, happiness and fulfilment of both refugees/newcomers and community population.

We believe that community outcomes will directly contribute in a soft and short time to the integration process of newcomers.

Project Ponton Process Schema

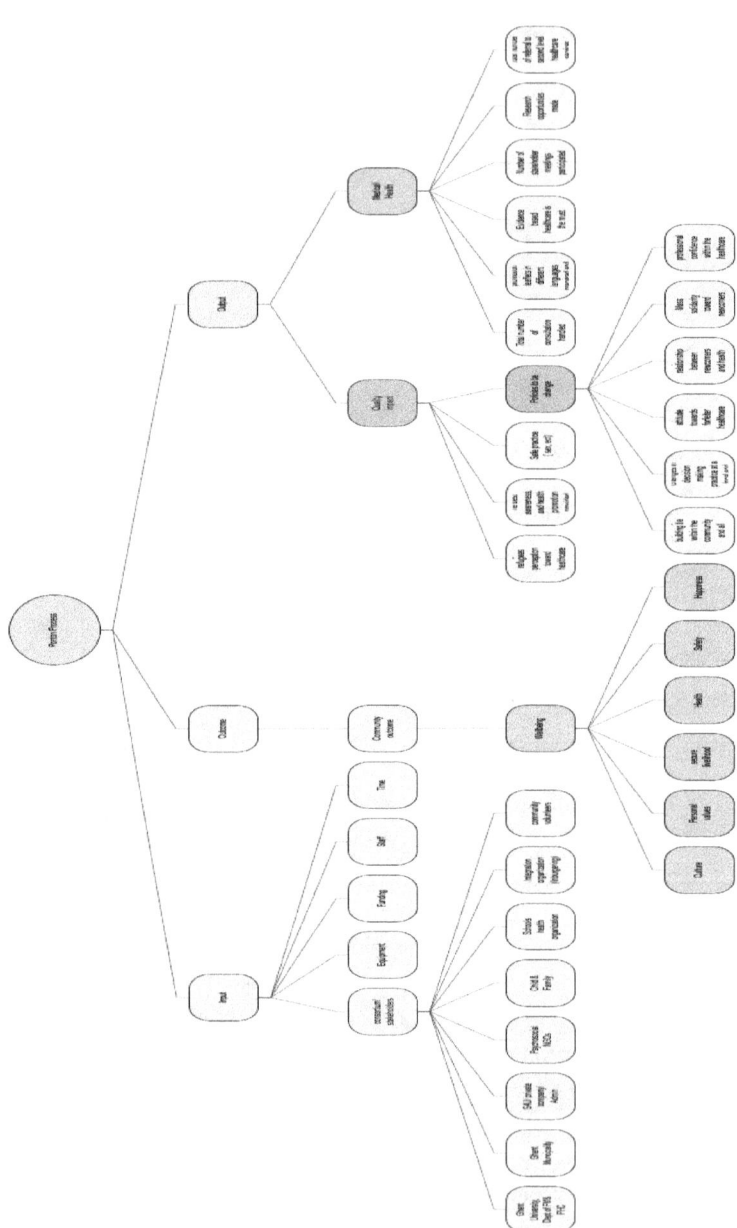

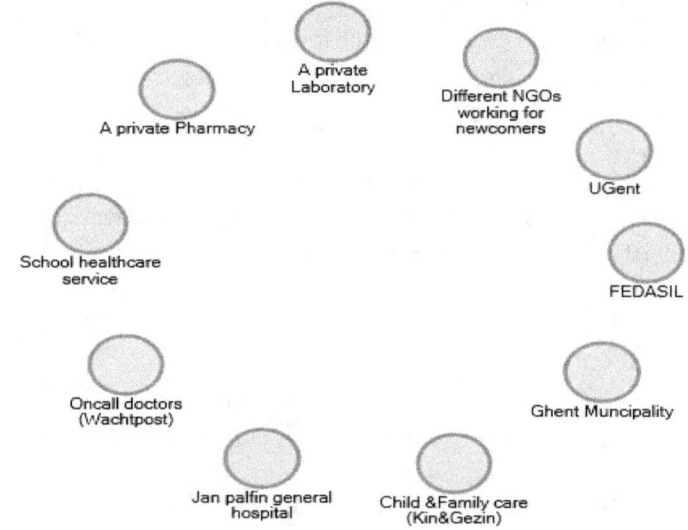

16, The main Ponton project healthcare stakeholders were:

1. FEDASIL[15]

2. Ghent University(Department of Family Medicine and Primary health care, department of Social Work) .

3. Ghent Municipality

4. Child &Family care(Kind&Gezin)

5. Jan Palfijn general hospital

6. On call doctors (Huisartsen wachtpost)

7. School healthcare service (CLB)

8. A private Pharmacy

9. A private Laboratory

10. Different NGOs working for and with Newcomers.

17. Enablers and barriers

Enablers and barriers to the work during the implementation of the Project Ponton[c] varied from immediate colleagues behavior up to the stakeholders and from Pontonc' management to of individuals living on the Ponton.

The backbone point was how barriers should be managed and how we could be able to solve the problems and find solutions to the problems; it was nothing except the best leadership, good communication and evidence based healthcare services and we named it "Barriers Breakers".

18. Medical Record

Provision of hard or electronic copies of any relevant documentation produced; mainly our patients' medical record was essentials in standard practice.

Due to FEDASIL's rules and guidelines we have to report by paperwork only, so we had to preserve hard copies of medical records too.

It was our main objective to save and maintain all medical records in a real-time and online web-based software which was Pricare® in which enables to code all data based on ICPC 2 and ICD-10.

Pricare® was created as a modular software package tailored for community health centers and (multidisciplinary) group practices. It offers the following modules:

- Management of administrative patient data

- Management of medical patient data.

- Multidisciplinary Groups on agenda

- Invoicing module for the standard payment system.

- Reporting- analysis module.

These modules are developed in close cooperation with representatives of users.

All modules are bilingual French-Dutch, depending on the language of the user.

19. Qualitative impacts

Qualitative impacts are the less tangible progress toward our aim. Overall qualitative impacts in Pontonc' project achieved are:

a. Improved knowledge of refugees about healthcare system,

b. Health awareness and health promotion was provided

c. Improved community solidarity towards newcomers

d. Developed capability of building links within the community and with all players

e. Enhanced knowledge of refugees on safe practice (e.g. sex), bed buds prevention, body pain handling, physical exercises, sun exposure(Vit.D deficiency) and many more.

20. Conclusion and discussion

Exploring Asylum seekers[6'] medical, emotional and psychosocial needs and prepare them for a long term therapy is a fundamental issue and a challenge!

For the medical word, we realized that the presenting epidemiological aspects of diseases can be easily controlled by implementing comprehensive primary healthcare services, thus diagnosing, treating and preventing of the Scabies, Malaria, sexual transmitted diseases were an easy and systematic job. Beside offering different vaccines according to the guideline also counted as a huge strategic epidemiological intervention. Routine check-up and diagnosis and treatment of seasonal diseases along with avoiding unnecessary use of antibiotics was a tremendous job done by our team.

During our consultations we discovered that newcomers are facing feelings of being "different" and have "low" self-confidence. These differences made them internally and externally uncertain: internally they feel anxiety and fear and externally they placed on pressure through administration and employees of Asylum seekers[6] center to become so called a "reliable resident". The ethics of these interactions should be looked after carefully.

Putting 250 human in a boat who were for days or months on their way in water and fought for their lives probably not a good idea any more, despite of transforming prisoner boat to a river touched hotel as a residential place: Psychologically these people will remember those moments of their fight against salty heavy water in the oceans on their journey towards Europe.

All above together makes a newcomer an "outrageous creature" of the nature. Newcomers are mostly victims of the war, prosecution, torture, political unrest, poverty and the majority of them diagnosing for Post-Traumatic Stress Disorder (PTSD), the main sign and symptoms of PTSD are: upsetting memories, flashbacks, and nightmares, as well as feelings of distress or intense physical reactions when reminded of the event (e.g. sweating, pounding heart, nausea), stress, anxiety, sleeplessness, muscle and body pain. Based on evidence based medicine here in Belgium and Europe; the majority of newcomers showing signs and symptoms of PTSD, receive treatment for PTSD up to many years. We here in Ponton[c] have observed that due to an Acute incident of mental disorder which we suggested to name ATSD (Acquired Traumatic Stress Disorder) the newcomers might be double up their psychological illness which will have a negative impact on their health , integration and society as their big new family. There are many causes of ATSD such as: anxiety and fear from the new environment among the newcomers, immoral integration process, cultural differences, a different eye on new comers as a different nature creature, inequity in health, high expectation from newcomers in a short time through host country, lower respect, "lower qualified person" mentality against highly educated newcomers, and many more enhancing newcomers' psychological problems balance negatively. So people easily can double their PTSD by ATSD.

In Ponton[c] we discovered Acquired Traumatic Stress Disorders (ASD) which was the main causes were uncertainty and long waiting time for getting status of refugee either rejecting their asylum appeal, feeling of being detainees, inappropriate communication through center personnel. Because of different and diverse culture, newcomers mostly don't talk about the causes , they reflect the causes by telling a symptom. The main reflecting symptoms were sleeplessness, anxiety, stress, headache, back pain, anger and self-harm.

We suggest that this model of short term interventions is a vital endeavor to identify and work with the Asylum seekers[6'] health needs, their resilience, strengths, positive assets, experience. We think it will be more feasible if we could be able to promote and adopt a follow up long term therapy model; this could help enormously for shortening and reducing of integration's time period in hosting country (Belgium).

To answer the question on equity in health and improvement health of newcomers we are in need of more studies.

21. Policy recommendation:

For a long term policy development and attainment of health equity and equality, we reached to propose the following:

More preparedness needed!

Preparedness means investment: Project Ponton[c] was not just a unique project to show our solidarity to the newcomers, but it became a fantastic lesson learned about the current situation of refugees in Belgium which lead to the following recommendations:

21.1 Infrastructure

Having an idea about immigration in the world which is not a new phenomenon and by predictions of scholars that rapidly the number of newcomers will be increasing in the coming years[2], we should prepare more by organizing standard infrastructure and preparing for receiving the newcomers even if it isn't our choice.

21.2 Training:

Prior knowledge of immigration and its consequences, knowledge about national and international law and regulations on refugees/Asylum seekers[6] and knowledge of basic psychology and intercultural and diversity communication skills will benefit newcomers to easily interact with hosts and integrate easily, smoothly and in a short term.

To provide comprehensive training on refugees and immigration to increase professional confidence working with newcomers both within the health and welfare providers and administrative workers is the must!

21.3 Political Deal

Dealing with a needy human-being is far away from political and religious believes; it's just a heart beating positive energy for help and hand giving to maintain and empower our human species every where in the globe.

We encourage politicians to follow international humanitarian agreement to bring changes in decision making practice towards providing standard healthcare services to refugees at a local and national levels.

21.4 Sustainability

We suggest that this model of short term interventions (Project Ponton[c]) is a vital endeavor to identify and work with the Asylum seekers[6'] health needs, resilience, strengths, positive assets, experience. We think it will be more feasible if we could be able to promote and adopt a follow up long term therapy model; hypothetically it may possibly help enormously for shortening and reducing of integration's time period in hosting country (Belgium).

21.5 Research

For a better newcomers/ refugees care management in the future and its sustainability, the Project Ponton[c] lessons learned may escort interested governmental and non-governmental bodies toward more understanding and the undertaking of relevant research for equity in refugees health.

Refugees and Asylum seekers[6] are mostly ignored in health policy, data and research. While many health issues are ignored as an area of integration policy. Scholars and cultural insiders who can touch and handle the level of complexity involved in doing research on refugees, should come across of this kind of research, they should be able to make possible any code of ethics and successfully resolve the multiple ethical impasses that arise when doing research on refugees. Scientists involved in this kind of research should be fully familiar with the ethical issues and concerns of the migrant cultures, preferably scientists by an immigration background may be involved. In addition, researchers should devote sufficient time and resources to engage in the process of recruiting participants into the research project, obtaining truly informed consent, and assuring ethical communication with participants by offering diverse culturally accepted incentive to research participants.

22. Definitions
Asylum seekers Defination[6]

An asylum-seeker is someone whose request for sanctuary has yet to be processed. Every year, around one million or more people seek asylum.

National asylum systems are in place to determine who qualifies for international protection. However, during mass movements of refugees, usually as a result of conflict or violence, it is not always possible or necessary to conduct individual interviews with every asylum seeker who crosses a border. These groups are often called 'prima facie' refugees.

UNHCR believes that everyone has a right to seek asylum from persecution, and does its best to protect those who need it.[http://www.unhcr.org/asylum-seekers.html]

Refugee Definition[8]

In the United Nations' Convention of 1951, a refugee is more narrowly defined (in Article 1A) as a person who's "owing to a well-founded fear of being persecuted for reasons of race, religion, nationality, membership of a particular social group, or political opinion, is outside the country of his nationality, and is unable to or, owing to such fear, is unwilling to avail himself of the protection of that country". The concept of a refugee was expanded by the Convention's 1967 Protocol and by regional conventions in Africa and Latin America to include people who had fled war or other violence in their home country.

Primary health care (PHC)

PHC refers to the concept elaborated in the 1978 Declaration of Alma-Ata, which is based on the principles of equity, participation, intersectoral action, appropriate technology and a central role played by the health system.

Primary care (PC)

Primary care is more than just the level of care or gate keeping; it is a key process in the health system. It is first-contact, accessible, continued, comprehensive and coordinated care. First-contact care is accessible at the time of need; ongoing care focuses on the long-term health of a person rather than the short duration of the disease; comprehensive care is a range of services appropriate to the common problems in the respective population and coordination is the role by which primary care acts to coordinate other specialists that the patient may need. PC is a subset of PHC.

General practice

General practice is a term now often used loosely to cover the general practitioner and other personnel, and is therefore synonymous with primary care and family medicine. Originally, it was meant to describe the concept and model around the most significant single player in primary care: the general practitioner or primary care physician, while family medicine originally encompassed the notion of a team approach. Whenever the concept of solo practitioner (general practice) versus team -based approach (family medicine) is relevant, the distinction is still made (and important). The specificity of the general practitioner is that he/she is: "the only clinician who operates at the nine levels of care: prevention, pre-symptomatic detection of disease, early diagnosis, diagnosis of established disease, management of disease, management of disease complications, rehabilitation, palliative care and counselling". [Atun R. What are the advantages and disadvantages of restructuring a health care system to be more focused on primary care services, WHO/Europe, 2004]

Family medicine (FM) or primary care

Family medicine (FM) or primary care teams can vary between countries and in size, the core team usually is the general practitioner and a nurse, but can comprise a multidisciplinary team of up to 30 professionals including community nurses, midwives, feldshers, dentists, physiotherapists, social workers, psychiatrists, speech therapists, dietitians, pharmacists, administrative staff and managers. In 2003, WHO defined a primary care team as a group of "fellow professionals with complementary contributions to make in patient care. This would be part of a broader social trend away from deference and hierarchy and towards mutual respect and shared responsibility and cooperation". By definition primary care/family medicine teams are patient centered, so their composition and organizational model can change over time.

Comprehensive Primary Healthcare

Comprehensive Primary Healthcare (CPHC)[1] is a framework considered as a global strategy to reduce inequities in health between and within nations and emphasizing the community action. The aims through Project Ponton intervention remain: refugees' equitable access to care, community participation, devotion to social determinants of health, intersectoral cooperations and health advocacy.

23. References

1. EUROPEAN CIVIL PROTECTION AND HUMANITARIAN AID OPERATIONS http://ec.europa.eu/echo/refugee-crisis_en

2. https://stad.gent/ghent-international

3. http://site.figac.be/pricare-nl.asp

4. http://www.ugent.be/ge/primarycare/en

5. https://stad.gent/samenleven-welzijn-gezondheid/diverse-stad/asiel-en-vluchtelingen/solidair-gent/privaat-opvangcentrum-voor-asielzoekers-aan-de-rigakaai-reno

6. http://www.unhcr.org/asylum-seekers.html

1. 7. Boano et al. 2008, Brown 2007, UNHCR 2009 http://ehp.niehs.nih.gov/wp-content/uploads/120/5/ehp.1104375.pdf

8. UNHCR: http://www.unhcr.org/refugees.html

9. http://www.unhcr.org/4ec262df9.pdf

10. https://www.globalhealthequity.ca/content/comprehensive-primary-health-care

11. https://www.semanticscholar.org/paper/What-are-the-advantages-and-disadvantages-of-Atun/5258e155e8d63943537b6716153b97406211d8f7

12. https://www.ncbi.nlm.nih.gov/pmc/articles/PMC1692964/pdf/12028796.pdf

13. http://www.unrefugees.org/what-is-a-refugee/

14. http://www.unhcr.org/asylum-seekers.html

15. http://fedasil.be/en Fedral agency for reception of Asylum seekers6

16. http://ec.europa.eu/eurostat/statistics-explained/index.php/Healthcare_activities_statistics_-_consultations

17. http://www.huisvoorgezondheid.be/patient/de-mutualiteit

18. a-General practitioners ,

19. b- Federal Agency for the Reception od Asylum seekers,

20. c- Name of Asylum Seekers Center in Ghent